FOREVER YOUNG DIET COOKBOOK 2024

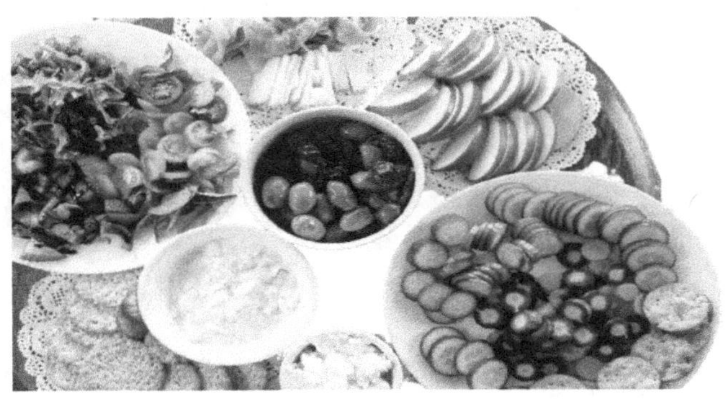

With this meticulously crafted collection of recipes, you can improve your health and embrace a vibrant

Misty J. Font

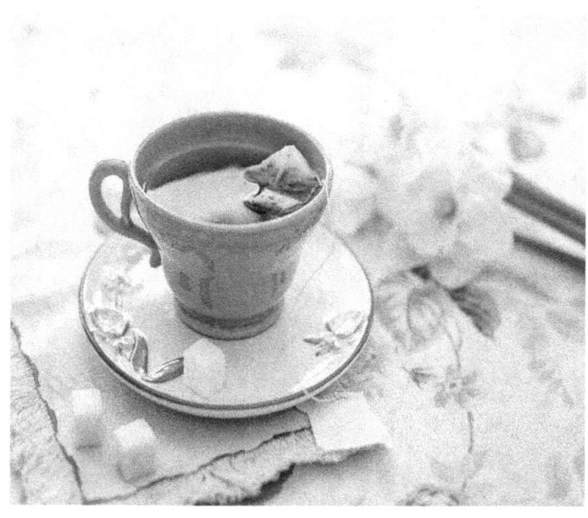

Table of content

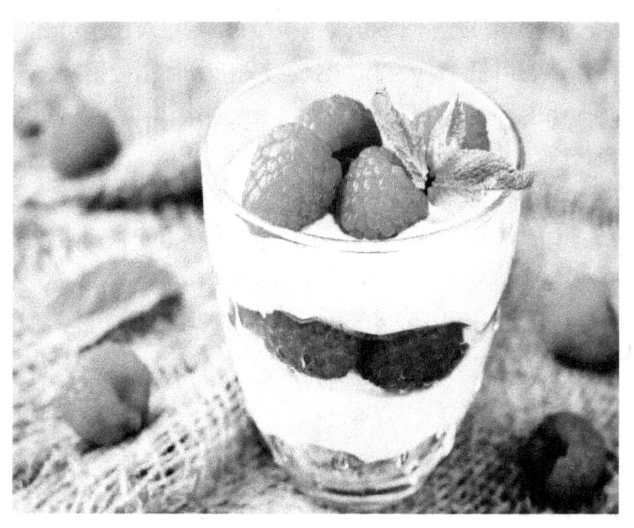

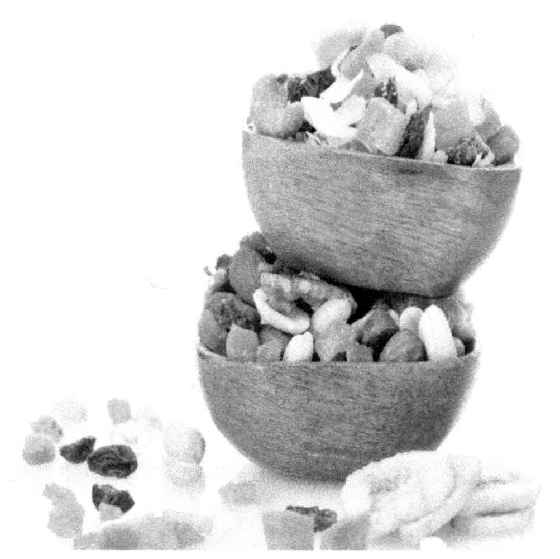

INTRODUCTION

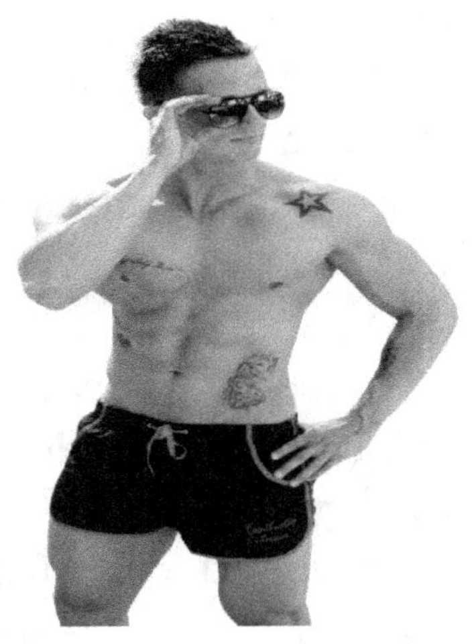

the curious town of Evergreen Springs, settled between moving slopes and a prattling creek, carried on with a man named Gerrard who appeared to resist the ways of the world. His brilliant energy and energetic shine were all the rage, leaving local people fascinated and pondering the mysterious behind his unending essentialness.

Gerrard, an unassuming and pleasant person, had consumed his time on earth embracing a way of thinking that rose above the traditional comprehension of maturing. At the core of his immortal process was the "Eternity Youthful Eating regimen Cookbook," a culinary book of scriptures that had turned into his confided in sidekick chasing timeless youth.

Gerrard's journey to eternal vitality began when he found the cookbook among the dusty books in the charming town bookstore. Attracted to its promising title and lively cover, he flipped through the pages, finding a gold mine of recipes and nourishing experiences that reverberated with his craving for a better, more dynamic life.

As Gerrard dove into the cookbook's pages, he found an assortment of recipes as well as a comprehensive manual for supporting the body and soul. The cookbook, composed by famous sustenance specialists, divulged the science behind the maturing system and the significant effect that nourishment could have on dialing it back. Gerrard, ever the energetic student, ingested the information like a wipe, anxious to apply it to his own life.

The cookbook acquainted Gerrard with a universe of supplement rich fixings, hostile to maturing superfoods, and shrewd cooking procedures that guaranteed flavorful feasts as well as a way to supported essentialness. It turned into his compass, directing him through the making of dinners that were as satisfying to the taste buds as they were useful to his general prosperity.

One of Gerrard's #1 recipes from the cookbook was the "Quinoa Power Porridge" that he enjoyed each day. Loaded with protein, fiber, and a horde of nutrients, this morning meal bowl turned into the foundation of his day. As he enjoyed every spoonful, he could feel the energy flowing through his veins, prepared to handle anything challenges the day introduced.

The "Eternity Youthful Eating routine Cookbook" turned into Gerrard's culinary compatriot, going with him through different sections of his life. From the dynamic "Invigorating Smoothie Bowls" that filled his mornings to the soothing "Rainbow Plates of mixed greens Overflowing with Cancer prevention agents" that graced his snacks, the cookbook's recipes decorated his table, changing dinners into customs of sustenance and taking care of oneself.

As Gerrard embraced the cookbook's lessons, he didn't simply take on a bunch of recipes; he embraced a way of life. The cookbook had an impact that went beyond the kitchen. It taught him to choose restaurants with care, helped him select a selection of portable snacks for his outdoor adventures, and even inspired him to create signature cocktails at his social gatherings that were both indulgent and beneficial to his health.

The townsfolk wondered about Gerrard's ever-enduring appearance and irresistible vitality, and soon, murmurs of the "Eternity Youthful Eating routine Cookbook" spread like quickly. It turned into a wellspring of motivation for the overwhelming majority, changing Evergreen Springs into a local area that esteemed the progression of time as well as the nature of the excursion.

The transformational power of adopting a lifestyle based on the principles of the "Forever Young Diet Cookbook" is demonstrated by Gerrard's story. As he proceeded with his excursion through the embroidery of life, Gerrard turned into a living encapsulation of the cookbook's commitment — an immortal demonstration of the significant effect that cognizant and feeding decisions can have on the quest for never-ending youth

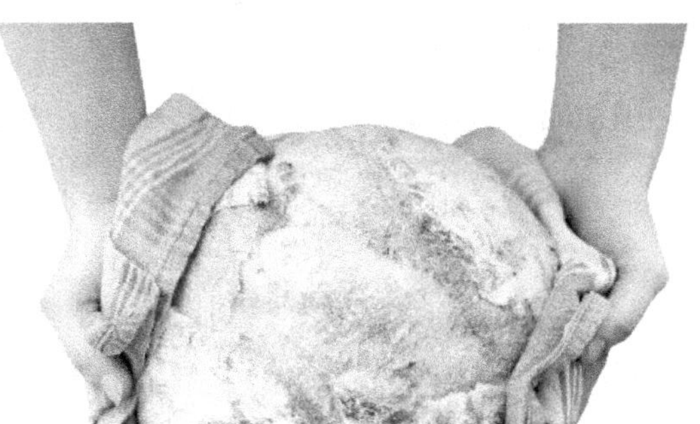

CHAPTER 1: THE WELLSPRING OF YOUTH IN YOUR PLATE

In the clamoring ensemble of present day life, our plates have become more than simple wellsprings of food; We can gain access to the elixir of eternal vitality through them. Welcome to Section 1 of the "Eternity Youthful Food" cookbook, where we set out on a culinary investigation to reveal the Wellspring of Youth that exists in the domain of our everyday feasts.

Investigating Against Maturing Superfoods

Our process starts with a journey for the unprecedented — nature's gift to us as hostile to maturing superfoods. These healthful forces to be reckoned with are not simply fixings; they are chemists of wellbeing, working synergistically to restore and rejuvenate our bodies. From the energetic shades of cell reinforcement rich berries to the omega-3 unsaturated fats found in greasy fish, we dig into the different universe of superfoods that battle the desolates of time.

Plan to find how integrating these culinary diamonds into your eating regimen can intensify your body's strength, battle irritation, and give a characteristic safeguard against the mileage of day to day existence. Through tempting recipes and keen tips, we guide you on a gastronomic odyssey, making hostile to maturing sustenance an extravagance as opposed to an errand.

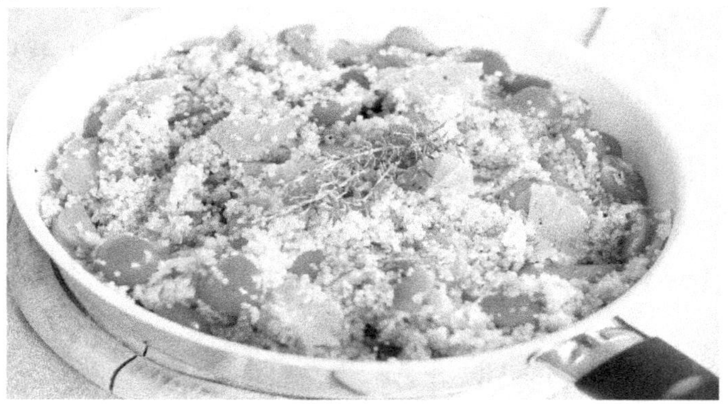

The Power of Nutrient-Packed Ingredients Beyond the allure of superfoods are the essential components of longevity—nutrient-packed ingredients that serve as the foundation for our culinary creations. In this part, we disentangle the wholesome orchestra inside every fixing, investigating the nutrients, minerals, and phytonutrients that add to the concordance of a very much supported body.

Learn about the transformative properties of leafy greens, legumes' prowess as a source of protein, and colorful vegetables' enchantment with micronutrients. We demystify the healthful profiles of regular fixings, enabling you to pursue informed decisions that entice your taste buds as well as sustain your body from the inside.

How Different Food Groups Help You Stay Younger
Your plate is like a canvas, and the choices you make when putting it together will make or break your health. This segment discloses the imaginativeness of young living by analyzing how different nutritional categories add to the orchestra of prosperity. From the essentialness helping characteristics of lean proteins to the energy-rich hug of entire grains, we guide you through the different range of nutritional categories that structure the range old enough resisting nourishment.

Get ready to develop a plate that isn't simply a variety of flavors yet an all encompassing piece intended to feed and support. Understanding the roles that carbohydrates, fats, and proteins play in promoting sustained energy, mental clarity, and physical resilience helps you find balance.

As you set out on this gastronomic undertaking, let every recipe be a brushstroke, painting a dynamic embroidery of prosperity. The Wellspring of Youth is certainly not a legendary spring yet a rich and different cluster of fixings ready to be relished. Go along with us in Section 1 as we open the mysteries of ever-enduring living, each delightful chomp in turn.

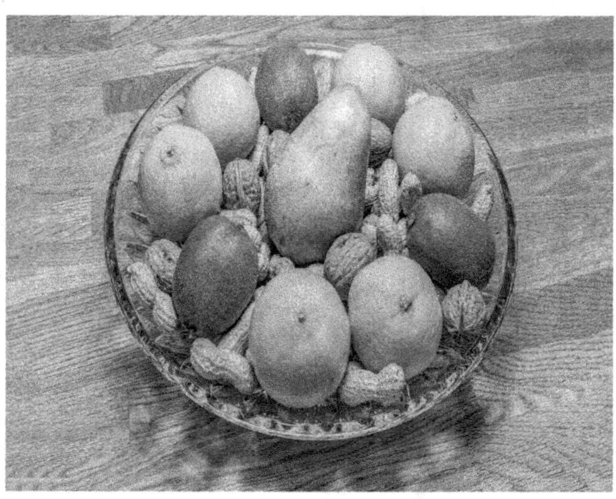

CHAPTER 2: MAKING A KITCHEN THAT STAYS YOUNG FOREVER

The kitchen is a haven for health, vitality, and culinary creativity in every home. Your guide to creating a kitchen that not only echoes with the sizzle of healthy meals but also serves as the workshop for your journey toward enduring well-being is found in Chapter 2 of the cookbook "Forever Young Cuisine."

Loading Up on Fundamental Fixings

Step into a kitchen that serves as a mother lode of wellbeing. This segment is your visa to the universe of fundamental fixings, cautiously arranged to imbue your dinners with the lavishness of supplements and the energy of flavors. From the storage space staples that structure the foundation old enough challenging recipes to the new produce that reinvigorates your culinary manifestations, we investigate the craft of loading up on fixings that support both body and soul.

Plan to change your kitchen into a material where each flavor, each grain, and each spice adds to the show-stopper of your prosperity. As you leave on this investigation, think of it as a shopping list as well as a statement for a way of life that values the job of food as medication.

Must-Have Kitchen Instruments for Easy Solid Cooking

Easy solid cooking starts with the right instruments. The essentials that will transform your kitchen into a haven of culinary efficiency are revealed in this section. From accuracy cuts that dance through vegetables to shrewd machines that smooth out your cooking cycle, we guide you through the fundamental munititions stockpile that each Eternity Youthful Kitchen ought to brag.

Find how the right devices save time as well as improve the healthy benefit of your feasts. We demystify the universe of kitchen contraptions, guaranteeing that every thing fills a need in advancing a way of life of straightforwardness and health. Let the bang of pots and the murmur of blenders be the soundtrack to your excursion towards an eternity youthful you.

Efficient Dinner Prep Tips for Occupied Ways of life

In the tornado of current life, time is a valuable product. This part is your compass to explore the requests of a bustling timetable without settling for less on your obligation to wellbeing. You can live the Forever Young Lifestyle without feeling tethered to the stove by following our time-saving meal preparation tips.

From vital clump cooking to productive capacity arrangements, we engage you to pursue wellbeing cognizant decisions even on the most active of days. As you integrate these tips into your daily practice, let dinner readiness become a careful custom instead of an overwhelming undertaking.

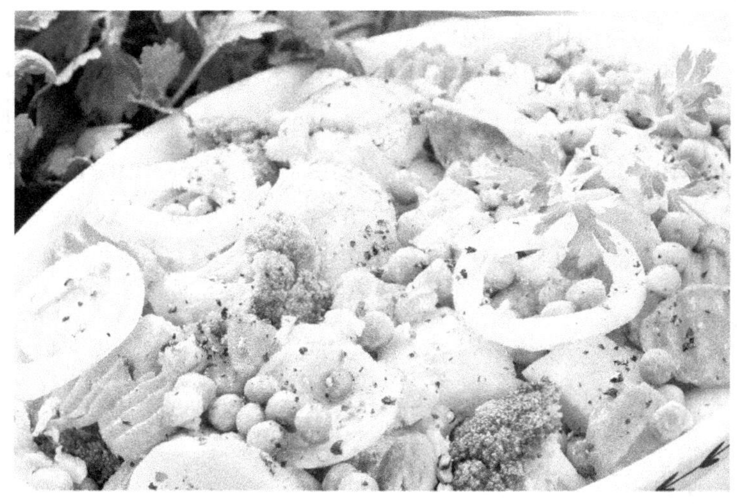

A Forever Young Kitchen is more than just putting together tools and ingredients; it's tied in with mixing your culinary space with goal, delight, and the expectation of feeding both yourself and your friends and family. In Chapter 2, we'll take you on a practical yet profound journey to design a kitchen that reflects the vitality you seek in your daily life. Join us as we begin this journey.

CHAPTER 3: BREAKFASTS CHAMPIONS

Sunrise Smoothie Bowl

Brief Description/Backstory: Start your day with a burst of energy and a riot of colours. This Sunrise Smoothie Bowl is not only delicious but also visually appealing. It's a great way to start the day because it's high in antioxidants and vitamins.

Serving Size: 2
Prep Time & Cooking Time: 10 minutes

Ingredients:
- 2 frozen bananas
- 1 cup mixed berries (strawberries, blueberries, raspberries)
- 1 cup mango chunks
- 1 cup spinach leaves
- 1 cup almond milk
- 2 tablespoons chia seeds

Toppings:

- sliced kiwi,
- granola, coconut flakes, and a drizzle of honey

Instructions:
1. Blend frozen bananas, mixed berries, mango chunks, spinach, and almond milk in a blender.
2. Blend until the mixture is smooth and creamy.
3. Pour the smoothie into serving bowls.
4. Served with sliced kiwi, granola, coconut flakes, and honey drizzle.
5. Take pleasure in the vibrant flavours and nourishing goodness.

Quinoa Power Porridge

Brief Description/Backstory: This Quinoa Power Porridge is a protein-packed alternative to traditional oats that will improve your morning routine. It's the ultimate breakfast for champions, with a delightful nutty flavour and a creamy texture that will fuel your day with sustained energy.

Serving Size: 4
Prep Time & Cooking Time: 15 minutes

Ingredients:
- 1 cup quinoa, rinsed
- 2 cups almond milk
- 1 teaspoon vanilla extract
- 1/4 cup chopped nuts (almonds, walnuts, or your choice)
- 2 tablespoons maple syrup
- Fresh berries for topping

Instructions:
1. Combine the quinoa, almond milk, and vanilla extract in a saucepan.
2. Bring to a boil, then reduce to a low heat, cover, and leave to cook for 12-15 minutes, or until the quinoa is tender and the mixture is creamy.
3. Add the chopped nuts and maple syrup and mix well.
4. Serve the porridge in bowls with fresh berries on top.
5. Enjoy the hearty goodness of this protein-packed breakfast.

Veggie-Packed Omelette Delight

Brief Description/Backstory: The Veggie-Packed Omelette Delight is a colourful and nutrient-dense dish that combines the goodness of eggs with a medley of vibrant vegetables. It's a savoury delight that will get your day started on a flavorful note.

Serving Size: 2
Prep Time & Cooking Time: 15 minutes

Ingredients:
- 4 large eggs
- 1/4 cup diced bell peppers (red, yellow, green)
- 1/4 cup cherry tomatoes, halved
- 1/4 cup spinach, chopped
- 1/4 cup feta cheese, crumbled
- Salt and pepper to taste
- 1 tablespoon olive oil

Instructions:
1. In a mixing bowl, whisk together the eggs and season with salt and pepper.
2. In a skillet over medium heat, heat the olive oil.

3. Cook until the diced bell peppers soften.
4. Over the vegetables in the skillet, pour the beaten eggs.
5. Distribute the cherry tomatoes, spinach, and feta cheese evenly over the eggs.
6. Cook until the edges are firm, then fold the omelette in half carefully.
7. Cook until the eggs have completely set.
8. Slide the omelette onto a plate and enjoy the delectable flavour combination.

Berry Blast Overnight Oats

Berry Blast Overnight Oats have a brief description/backstory that will help you have a stress-free morning. This dish combines ease of preparation with a burst of fruity flavours. You wake up to a delicious, ready-to-eat breakfast that fuels your day by soaking the oats overnight.

Serving Size: 2
Prep Time & Cooking Time: 5 minutes (plus overnight soaking)

Ingredients:

- 1 cup rolled oats
- 1 cup almond milk
- 1/2 cup mixed berries (strawberries, blueberries, raspberries)
- 2 tablespoons Greek yogurt
- 1 tablespoon honey
- 1/4 cup chopped nuts (e.g., almonds or walnuts)
- Fresh mint leaves for garnish

Instructions:

1. Combine rolled oats, almond milk, mixed berries, Greek yoghurt, and honey in a jar or bowl.
2. Refrigerate overnight after thoroughly mixing.
3. Stir the oats and top with chopped nuts in the morning.
4. Garnish with fresh mint leaves and serve your quick, nutrient-dense breakfast.

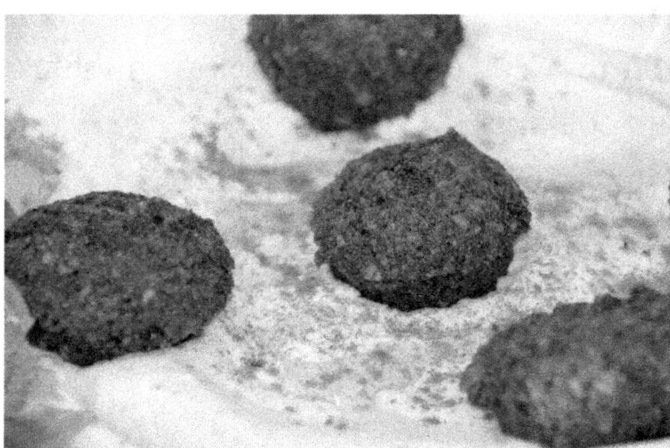

Avocado & Salmon Breakfast Toast

Brief Description/Backstory: The Avocado & Salmon Breakfast Toast is high in omega-3 fatty acids and other nutrients. This savoury delight not only pleases the palate but also provides a healthy balance of protein and fat.

Serving Size: 2
Prep Time & Cooking Time: 10 minutes

Ingredients:
- 4 slices whole-grain bread
- 1 ripe avocado, mashed
- 100g smoked salmon
- Cherry tomatoes, sliced
- Red onion, thinly sliced
- Fresh dill for garnish
- Lemon wedges for serving

Instructions:
1. Toast the slices of whole-grain bread.
2. Distribute the mashed avocado evenly on each slice.
3. Serve with smoked salmon, cherry tomatoes, and red onion on top.

4. Serve with lemon wedges on the side and garnished with fresh dill.

5. Enjoy the delectable combination of textures and flavours.

Sweet Potato and Spinach Breakfast Hash

Breif Description/Backstory: Sweet Potato and Spinach Breakfast Hash—a savoury and nutrient-dense medley of sweet potatoes, spinach, and eggs—will revitalise your mornings. This hearty dish contains the ideal combination of complex carbohydrates, fibre, and protein to keep you going throughout the day.

Serving Size: 2
Prep Time & Cooking Time: 20 minutes

Ingredients:
- 2 medium sweet potatoes, diced
- 2 cups fresh spinach
- 1 red bell pepper, diced
- 1 onion, finely chopped

- 2 eggs
- Olive oil for cooking
- Salt and pepper to taste
- Fresh herbs for garnish (e.g., parsley or chives)

Instructions:

1. Warm the olive oil in a skillet over medium heat.
2. Cook until the diced sweet potatoes begin to brown.
3. Sauté the diced red bell pepper and onion until softened.
4. Cook until the spinach has wilted.
5. Make two wells in the hash, one for each egg.
6. Cook, covered, until the eggs are done to your liking.
7. Season with salt and pepper, then top with fresh herbs and enjoy the hearty goodness.

Nutty Banana Pancakes

Brief Description/Backstory: Nutty Banana Pancakes will satisfy your taste buds and energise your morning. The sweetness of ripe bananas and the crunch of chopped nuts combine to create a delightful symphony of flavours in these light and fluffy pancakes.

Serving Size: 2-3
Prep Time & Cooking Time: 15 minutes

Ingredients:
- 1 cup all-purpose flour
- 1 tablespoon sugar
- 1 teaspoon baking powder
- 1/2 teaspoon baking soda
- 1/4 teaspoon salt
- 1 cup buttermilk
- 1 ripe banana, mashed
- 1 egg
- 2 tablespoons melted butter
- Chopped nuts (e.g., walnuts or pecans) for sprinkling
- Maple syrup for serving

Instructions:
1. In a mixing bowl, combine the flour, sugar, baking powder, baking soda, and salt.

2. In a separate mixing bowl, combine the buttermilk, mashed banana, egg, and melted butter.
3. Pour the wet ingredients into the dry ingredients and stir until just combined.
4. Warm a griddle or skillet over medium heat and lightly grease it.
5. For each pancake, pour 1/4 cup batter onto the griddle.
6. Before flipping each pancake, sprinkle with chopped nuts.
7. Cook until both sides are golden brown and serve with maple syrup.

Green Goddess Breakfast Wrap

Brief Description/Backstory: The Green Goddess Breakfast Wrap harnesses the power of greens. This wrap, filled with nutrient-rich spinach, avocado, and eggs, is a quick and portable breakfast that will give you a boost of energy to start your day.

Serving Size: 2
Prep Time & Cooking Time: 10 minutes

Ingredients:

- 4 whole-grain tortillas
- 4 large eggs
- 2 cups fresh spinach leaves
- 1 ripe avocado, sliced
- Cherry tomatoes, halved
- Feta cheese, crumbled
- Salt and pepper to taste
- Hot sauce for optional heat

Instructions:

1. Scramble the eggs in a skillet until done to your liking.
2. Heat the tortillas in a skillet or in the microwave.
3. Scrambled eggs, fresh spinach, avocado slices, cherry tomatoes, and crumbled feta cheese go into each wrap.
4. Season with salt and pepper, and if desired, add hot sauce.
5. Wrap the tortillas and enjoy the vibrant flavours on the go.

Mango Coconut Chia Pudding Bowl

Brief Description/Backstory: The Mango Coconut Chia Pudding Bowl will transport you to a tropical paradise. This exotic and refreshing breakfast is a harmonious blend of creamy coconut, luscious mango, and nutrient-rich chia seeds—a tropical taste to energise your morning routine.

Serving Size: 2
Prep Time & Cooking Time: 10 minutes (plus chilling time)

Ingredients:
- 1/4 cup chia seeds
- 1 cup coconut milk
- 1 ripe mango, diced
- 2 tablespoons shredded coconut
- 1 tablespoon honey or agave syrup
- Fresh mint leaves for garnish

Instructions:
1. Combine chia seeds and coconut milk in a mixing bowl. Allow it to sit for 5 minutes before stirring again to prevent clumping.

2. Refrigerate the mixture for at least 2 hours or overnight, or until it has the consistency of custard.
3. In bowls, alternate layers of chia pudding with diced mango and shredded coconut.
4. Drizzle with honey or agave syrup.
5. Garnish with fresh mint leaves and enjoy this nutritious breakfast bowl's tropical bliss.

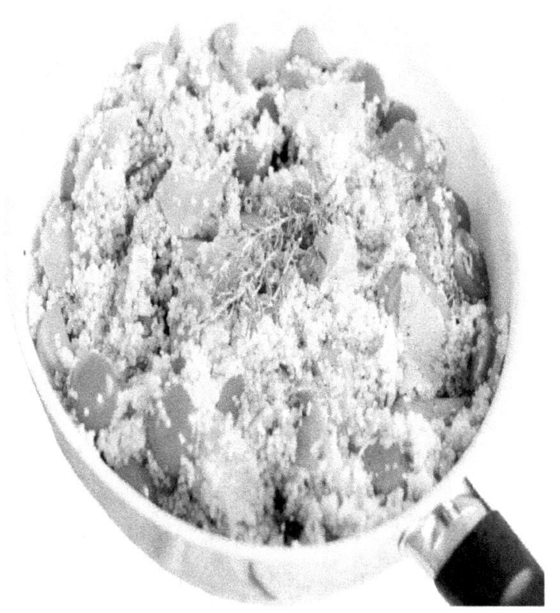

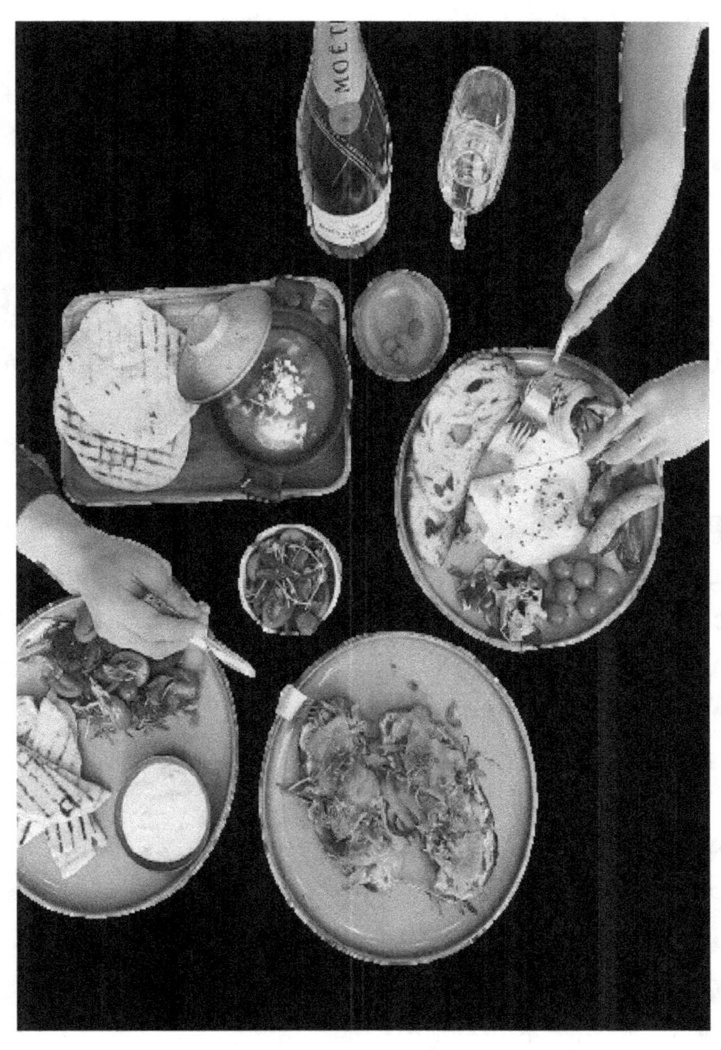

CHAPTER 4:NOURISHING LUNCHES FOR LASTING ENERGY

Vibrant Quinoa and Chickpea Rainbow Salad

Brief Description/Backstory: This Vibrant Quinoa and Chickpea Rainbow Salad—a symphony of colours, textures, and flavors—will elevate your lunchtime experience. This salad, which is high in nutrients, not only nourishes your body but also tantalises your taste buds.

Serving Size: 4
Prep Time & Cooking Time: 20 minutes

Ingredients:
- 1 cup cooked quinoa
- 1 can (15 oz) chickpeas, drained and rinsed
- 1 cup cherry tomatoes, halved
- 1 cucumber, diced

- 1 bell pepper (red or yellow), diced
- 1/2 red onion, finely chopped
- 1/4 cup Kalamata olives, sliced
- Feta cheese, crumbled
- Fresh parsley, chopped
- Olive oil, lemon juice, salt, and pepper for the dressing

Instructions:

1. Combine cooked quinoa, chickpeas, cherry tomatoes, cucumber, bell pepper, red onion, and Kalamata olives in a large mixing bowl.
2. In a small mixing bowl, combine the olive oil, lemon juice, salt, and pepper to taste. Drizzle the dressing over the salad and toss to combine.
3. Garnish the salad with crumbled feta cheese and fresh parsley.
4. For a filling and energising lunch, try this nutrient-dense rainbow delight.

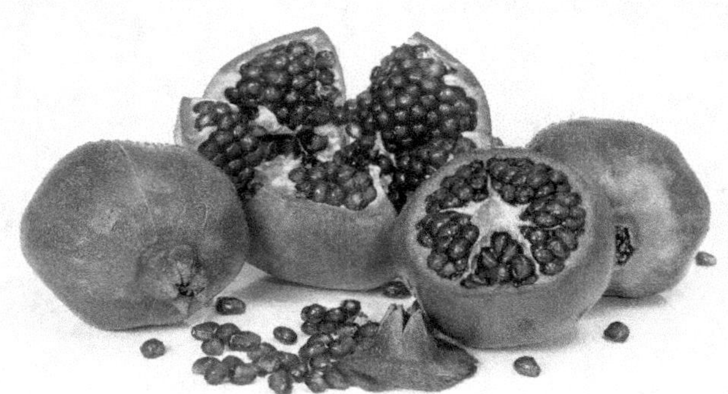

Teriyaki Chicken and Broccoli Power Bowl

Brief Description/Backstory: Power up your afternoon with the Teriyaki Chicken and Broccoli Power Bowl, a well-balanced combination of lean protein, vibrant vegetables, and flavorful teriyaki sauce. This bowl not only tastes good, but it also gives you energy for the rest of the day.

Serving Size: 2
Prep Time & Cooking Time: 25 minutes

Ingredients:
- 2 boneless, skinless chicken breasts, sliced
- 2 cups broccoli florets
- 1 red bell pepper, sliced
- 1 carrot, julienned
- 1 cup cooked brown rice
- Sesame seeds and green onions for garnish
- For the Teriyaki Sauce:
- 1/4 cup soy sauce
- 2 tablespoons honey
- 1 tablespoon rice vinegar
- 1 teaspoon sesame oil

- 1 teaspoon cornstarch mixed with 1 tablespoon water

Instructions:
1. To make the teriyaki sauce, whisk together the soy sauce, honey, rice vinegar, sesame oil, and cornstarch-water mixture in a mixing bowl.
2. Cook sliced chicken in a skillet until browned.
3. Combine broccoli, red bell pepper, and julienned carrot in a mixing bowl. Cook until the vegetables are soft.
4. Serve the chicken and vegetables with the teriyaki sauce. Stir to ensure an even coating.
5. Over cooked brown rice, serve the teriyaki chicken and vegetables.
6. Serve with sesame seeds and green onions as garnish. Take pleasure in the flavorful and protein-rich power bowl.

Mediterranean Chickpea and Quinoa Wrap

Brief Description/Backstory: The Mediterranean Chickpea and Quinoa Wrap is a delightful fusion of Mediterranean flavours wrapped in a whole-grain tortilla. This portable lunch option provides you with long-lasting energy on the go.

Serving Size: 2
Prep Time & Cooking Time: 15 minutes

Ingredients:
- 1 cup cooked quinoa
- 1 can (15 oz) chickpeas, drained and rinsed
- 1 cup cherry tomatoes, halved
- 1 cucumber, sliced
- 1/4 cup red onion, thinly sliced
- Feta cheese, crumbled
- Kalamata olives, sliced
- Hummus for spreading
- Whole-grain tortillas

Instructions:

1. Combine cooked quinoa, chickpeas, cherry tomatoes, cucumber, red onion, crumbled feta, and sliced Kalamata olives in a mixing bowl.
2. On each whole-grain tortilla, spread hummus.
3. Fill the tortillas with the quinoa and chickpea mixture.
4. Fold the wraps in half and roll them up.
5. Cut in half and secure with toothpicks if necessary.
6. On the go, enjoy the Mediterranean goodness.

Asian-Inspired Tofu and Vegetable Stir-Fry

Brief Description/Backstory: Savour the Asian-Inspired Tofu and Vegetable Stir-Fry, a quick and flavorful lunch option that combines the goodness of tofu with a colourful array of crisp vegetables.

Serving Size: 3
Prep Time & Cooking Time: 20 minutes

Ingredients:

- 1 block extra-firm tofu, pressed and cubed
- 2 cups broccoli florets
- 1 red bell pepper, sliced
- 1 carrot, julienned
- 1 cup snap peas, ends trimmed
- 3 tablespoons soy sauce
- 1 tablespoon hoisin sauce
- 1 tablespoon sesame oil
- 1 tablespoon rice vinegar
- 2 cloves garlic, minced
- 1 teaspoon ginger, grated
- Cooked brown rice for serving

Instructions:

1. Heat sesame oil in a wok or skillet over medium-high heat. Cook until the tofu cubes are golden brown. Set aside the tofu from the pan.
2. If necessary, add a little more sesame oil to the same pan. Broccoli, red bell pepper, carrot, and snap peas should be sautéed until crisp-tender.

3. Whisk together soy sauce, hoisin sauce, rice vinegar, minced garlic, and grated ginger in a small bowl.
4. Pour the sauce over the tofu and vegetables after adding the cooked tofu back to the pan. Toss until thoroughly coated.
5. Serve the stir-fry of tofu and vegetables over cooked brown rice. For long-lasting energy, eat this savoury and nutritious lunch.

Quinoa and Black Bean Stuffed Peppers

Brief Description/Backstory: Quinoa and Black Bean Stuffed Peppers—a wholesome and protein-packed dish that combines the goodness of quinoa, black beans, and a medley of flavorful vegetables—will revitalise your lunchtime.

Serving Size: 4
Prep Time & Cooking Time: 30 minutes

Ingredients:
- 4 large bell peppers, halved and seeds removed

- 1 cup cooked quinoa
- 1 can (15 oz) black beans, drained and rinsed
- 1 cup corn kernels (fresh or frozen)
- 1 cup diced tomatoes
- 1/2 cup red onion, finely chopped
- 1 teaspoon ground cumin
- 1 teaspoon chili powder
- Salt and pepper to taste
- Shredded cheese for topping (optional)
- Fresh cilantro for garnish

Instructions:

1. Preheat the oven to 375 degrees Fahrenheit (190 degrees Celsius).
2. Combine cooked quinoa, black beans, corn, diced tomatoes, red onion, ground cumin, chilli powder, salt and pepper in a large mixing bowl.
3. Fill each halved bell pepper half with the quinoa mixture.
4. Cover the stuffed peppers in a baking dish with foil.

Salmon and Avocado Sushi Bowl

Brief Description/Backstory: The Salmon and Avocado Sushi Bowl brings the essence of sushi to your lunchtime. This deconstructed sushi bowl combines the richness of salmon with the creaminess of avocado, providing a burst of flavours as well as Omega-3 fatty acids for long-lasting energy.

Serving Size: 2
Prep Time & Cooking Time: 15 minutes

Ingredients:
- 2 cups cooked sushi rice
- 200g fresh salmon, sashimi-grade, sliced
- 1 avocado, sliced
- 1 cucumber, julienned
- 2 sheets nori (seaweed), torn into strips
- 1 tablespoon soy sauce
- 1 tablespoon sesame oil
- Pickled ginger and wasabi for serving

Instructions:
1. Serve the cooked sushi rice in two bowls.

2. On top of the rice, layer sliced salmon, avocado, cucumber, and nori strips.
3. Drizzle with sesame oil and soy sauce.
4. On the side, serve with pickled ginger and wasabi.

Salmon and Avocado Sushi Bowl

Brief Description/Backstory: The Salmon and Avocado Sushi Bowl brings the essence of sushi to your lunchtime. This deconstructed sushi bowl combines the richness of salmon with the creaminess of avocado, providing a burst of flavours as well as Omega-3 fatty acids for long-lasting energy.

Serving Size: 2
Prep Time & Cooking Time: 15 minutes

Ingredients:
- 2 cups cooked sushi rice
- 200g fresh salmon, sashimi-grade, sliced
- 1 avocado, sliced
- 1 cucumber, julienned

- 2 sheets nori (seaweed), torn into strips
- 1 tablespoon soy sauce
- 1 tablespoon sesame oil
- Pickled ginger and wasabi for serving

Instructions:
1. Serve the cooked sushi rice in two bowls.
2. On top of the rice, layer sliced salmon, avocado, cucumber, and nori strips.
3. Drizzle with sesame oil and soy sauce.
4. On the side, serve with pickled ginger and wasabi.
5. Enjoy the pleasures of sushi flavours in a convenient and nourishing bowl.

Spicy Shrimp and Quinoa Stuffed Bell Peppers

Brief Description/Backstory: These Spicy Shrimp and Quinoa Stuffed Bell Peppers will liven up your lunch routine. Stuffed peppers with protein-rich prawns, quinoa and a zesty kick make for a filling and energising midday meal.

Serving Size: 4
Prep Time & Cooking Time: 35 minutes

Ingredients:
- 4 large bell peppers, halved and seeds removed
- 1 cup cooked quinoa
- 200g shrimp, peeled and deveined
- 1 cup black beans, drained and rinsed
- 1 cup corn kernels (fresh or frozen)
- 1/2 cup red onion, finely chopped
- 1 teaspoon cumin
- 1 teaspoon chili powder
- 1/2 teaspoon cayenne pepper (adjust to taste)
- Salt and pepper to taste
- Fresh cilantro for garnish

Instructions:
1. Preheat the oven to 375 degrees Fahrenheit (190 degrees Celsius).
2. Cook prawns in a skillet until pink and opaque. Take off the heat and cut into bite-sized pieces.
3. Combine cooked quinoa, chopped shrimp, black beans, corn, red onion, cumin, chilli

powder, cayenne pepper, salt and pepper in a large mixing bowl.
4. Fill each half of a bell pepper with the quinoa and shrimp mixture.
5. Bake the stuffed peppers in a baking dish for 20-25 minutes, or until the peppers are tender.
6. Garnish with fresh cilantro and enjoy the spicy and nourishing flavours of this lunch.

Greek Chicken Souvlaki Salad

Brief Description/Backstory: The Greek Chicken Souvlaki Salad transports your taste buds to the Mediterranean, featuring succulent chicken, crisp vegetables, and a tangy Greek dressing.

Serving Size: 2
Prep Time & Cooking Time: 25 minutes

Ingredients:
- 2 boneless, skinless chicken breasts
- 1 teaspoon dried oregano
- 1 teaspoon garlic powder
- Salt and pepper to taste
- 2 cups mixed salad greens

- 1 cucumber, sliced
- 1 cup cherry tomatoes, halved
- 1/2 red onion, thinly sliced
- Feta cheese, crumbled
- Kalamata olives, sliced
- For the Greek Dressing:
- 3 tablespoons extra-virgin olive oil
- 1 tablespoon red wine vinegar
- 1 teaspoon Dijon mustard
- 1 teaspoon dried oregano
- Salt and pepper to taste

Instructions:

1. Season the chicken breasts with dried oregano, garlic powder, salt, and pepper.
2. Grill or pan-sear the chicken until done. Cut into strips.
3. Combine mixed salad greens, cucumber, cherry tomatoes, red onion, crumbled feta, and Kalamata olives in a large mixing bowl.
4. In a small mixing bowl, combine the ingredients for the Greek dressing.
5. Drizzle the Greek dressing over the salad and top with sliced chicken.
6. Toss gently to combine before serving this Mediterranean-inspired meal.

Lentil and Vegetable Curry Bowl

Brief Description/Backstory: Warm your soul with the Lentil and Vegetable Curry Bowl, a hearty and nourishing dish that combines protein-packed lentils, vibrant vegetables, and aromatic spices for a satisfying and flavorful lunch.

Serving Size: 4
Prep Time & Cooking Time: 30 minutes

Ingredients:
- 1 cup dry lentils, rinsed and drained
- 2 tablespoons curry powder
- 1 teaspoon ground cumin
- 1 teaspoon ground coriander
- 1/2 teaspoon turmeric
- 1 can (14 oz) coconut milk
- 1 cup vegetable broth
- 1 cup cauliflower florets
- 1 cup carrots, sliced
- 1 cup bell peppers, diced
- 1 cup spinach leaves
- Cooked basmati rice for serving

Instructions:

1. Combine dry lentils, curry powder, ground cumin, ground coriander, turmeric, coconut milk, and vegetable broth in a large pot.
2. Bring to a boil, then reduce to a low heat and cook for 15-20 minutes, or until the lentils are tender.
3. Combine the cauliflower, carrots, and bell peppers. Continue to cook until the vegetables are tender.
4. Cook until the spinach has wilted.
5. Serve the lentil and vegetable curry over cooked basmati rice.
6. Enjoy the warming comfort of this curry bowl.

Turkey and Quinoa Stuffed Zucchini Boats

Brief Description/Backstory: Turkey and Quinoa Stuffed Zucchini Boats are a filling and protein-packed lunch option. This recipe turns zucchini into vessels for a flavorful mixture of ground turkey, quinoa, and aromatic spices, creating a nutritious and filling midday meal.

Serving Size: 4
Prep Time & Cooking Time: 40 minutes

Ingredients:
- 4 medium-sized zucchini
- 1 pound ground turkey
- 1 cup cooked quinoa
- 1/2 cup onion, finely chopped
- 2 cloves garlic, minced
- 1 teaspoon ground cumin
- 1 teaspoon smoked paprika
- 1/2 teaspoon chili powder
- Salt and pepper to taste
- 1 cup tomato sauce
- Shredded mozzarella cheese for topping

Instructions:
1. Preheat the oven to 375 degrees Fahrenheit (190 degrees Celsius).
2. Cut each zucchini in half lengthwise.
3. To make boats, scoop out the centre.

4. Cook ground turkey in a skillet until browned.

5. Sauté the chopped onion and minced garlic until softened.

6. Cooked quinoa, ground cumin, smoked paprika, chilli powder, salt, and pepper are all good additions.

7. Fill each zucchini boat halfway with the turkey-quinoa mixture.Place the stuffed zucchini boats in the

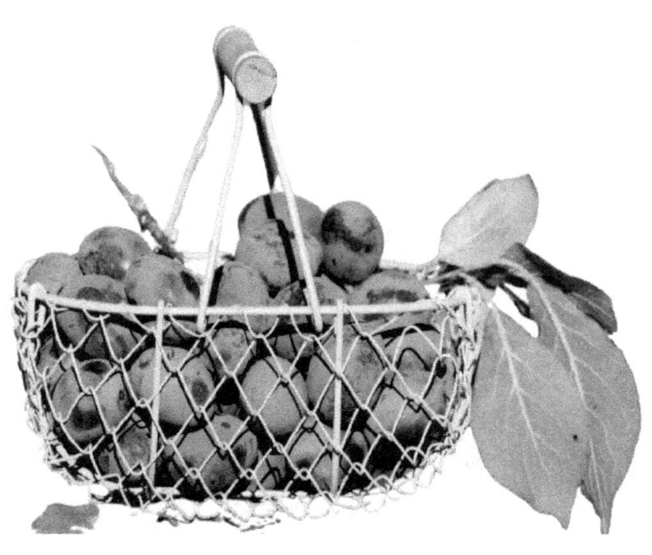

CHAPTER 5: DINNERS THAT DEFY AGE

Lemon Herb Baked Salmon with Quinoa Pilaf

Brief Description/Backstory: Lemon Herb Baked Salmon with Quinoa Pilaf is an elegant dish that combines the richness of salmon with the nuttiness of quinoa and a burst of citrusy herbs. This meal not only tempts the taste buds, but it also contains essential omega-3 fatty acids for a youthful glow.

Serving Size: 4
Prep Time & Cooking Time: 30 minutes

Ingredients:
- 4 salmon fillets
- 1 cup quinoa, rinsed
- 2 cups vegetable broth
- 1 lemon, thinly sliced
- Fresh parsley, chopped
- Olive oil

- Garlic powder, salt, and pepper to taste

Instructions:
1. Preheat the oven to 375 degrees Fahrenheit (190 degrees Celsius).
2. Garlic powder, salt, and pepper season salmon fillets.
3. Arrange the salmon fillets in a baking dish and surround with quinoa.
4. Pour the vegetable broth over the quinoa, then top with lemon slices.
5. Drizzle with olive oil and top with parsley.
6. Bake for 20-25 minutes, or until the salmon is cooked and the quinoa is tender, covered with foil.
7. Uncover and broil for 3-5 minutes more for a golden finish. Serve this culinary masterpiece with a side salad for an ageless dinner.

Mediterranean Stuffed Bell Peppers with Turkey

Brief Description/Backstory: These Stuffed Bell Peppers with a healthful blend of ground turkey, quinoa, tomatoes, and fragrant spices will transport your taste senses to the Mediterranean. This recipe not only represents the heart-healthy Mediterranean diet, but it also makes a filling and substantial dinner.

Serving Size: 4
Prep Time & Cooking Time: 40 minutes

Ingredients:
- 4 large bell peppers, halved and seeds removed
- 1 pound ground turkey
- 1 cup cooked quinoa
- 1 cup cherry tomatoes, diced
- 1/2 cup red onion, finely chopped
- 2 cloves garlic, minced
- 1 teaspoon dried oregano
- 1 teaspoon ground cumin
- Salt and pepper to taste
- Feta cheese for topping
- Fresh basil for garnish

Instructions:
1. Preheat the oven to 375 degrees Fahrenheit (190 degrees Celsius).

2. Cook ground turkey in a skillet until browned.

3. Sauté the red onion and garlic until tender.

4. Combine cooked quinoa, chopped cherry tomatoes, dried oregano, ground cumin, salt, and pepper in a large mixing bowl.

5. Fill each bell pepper half halfway with the turkey-quinoa mixture.

6. Place the filled peppers in a baking sheet, sprinkle with feta, and bake for 25-30 minutes, or until the peppers are soft.

7. Garnish with fresh basil and serve this age-defying Mediterranean-inspired supper.

Lentil and Vegetable One-Pot Curry

Brief Description/Backstory: The rich flavours of lentil and vegetable will delight your senses. One-Pot Curry is a plant-based meal that mixes protein-rich lentils with a variety of colourful veggies to create a dish that is as healthful as it is tasty.

Serving Size: 6

Prep Time & Cooking Time: 45 minutes

Ingredients:
- 1 cup dry lentils, rinsed and drained
- 2 tablespoons curry powder
- 1 teaspoon ground turmeric
- 1 teaspoon ground cumin
- 1 can (14 oz) coconut milk
- 1 cup vegetable broth
- 1 sweet potato, diced
- 1 cup cauliflower florets
- 1 cup green beans, trimmed
- 1 cup cherry tomatoes, halved
- 1 onion, diced
- 2 cloves garlic, minced
- Ginger, grated
- Olive oil
- Salt and pepper to taste
- Fresh cilantro for garnish

Instructions:
1. Heat the olive oil in a big saucepan and sauté the chopped onion until softened.
2. Stir in the minced garlic and grated ginger for another minute.

3. Stir in the curry powder, turmeric powder, and cumin powder.

4. Combine the dry lentils, sweet potato, cauliflower, green beans, cherry tomatoes, coconut milk, and vegetable broth in a mixing bowl.

5. Season with salt and pepper to taste.

6. Bring to a boil, then lower to a low heat and continue to cook for 30-35 minutes, or until the lentils and veggies are cooked.

7. For a filling meal, garnish with fresh cilantro and serve this flavorful curry over rice or quinoa.

Lemon Garlic Herb Grilled Chicken Breast

Brief Description/Backstory: Lemon Garlic Herb Grilled Chicken Breast is a recipe that combines the simplicity of grilled chicken with the freshness of lemon, the richness of garlic, and a fragrant combination of herbs. This protein-packed dish is ideal for people looking for a nutritious and satisfying evening.

Serving Size: 4
Prep Time & Cooking Time: 25 minutes

Ingredients:
- 4 boneless, skinless chicken breasts
- Zest and juice of 1 lemon
- 4 cloves garlic, minced
- Fresh herbs (rosemary, thyme, or oregano), chopped
- Olive oil
- Salt and pepper to taste

Instructions:
1. Combine lemon zest, lemon juice, minced garlic, chopped fresh herbs, olive oil, salt, and pepper in a mixing bowl.
2. Pour the marinade over the chicken breasts in a shallow dish. Allow for at least 15 minutes of marinating.
3. Preheat the grill to medium-high temperature.
4. Grill the chicken breasts for 6-8 minutes on each side.

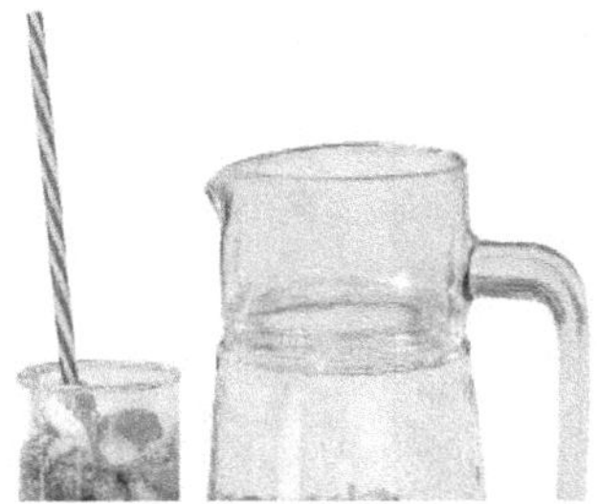

CHAPTER 6: SNACKING SMARTLY

Almond Butter and Banana Energy Bites

Brief Description/Backstory: Almond Butter and Banana Energy Bites are a delicious combination of healthful ingredients that deliver a burst of energy without the guilt. These bite-sized sweets will satisfy your sweet taste and keep you going throughout the day.

Serving Size: 12 bites
Prep Time & Cooking Time: 15 minutes (plus chilling time)

Ingredients:
- 1 cup rolled oats
- 1/2 cup almond butter
- 1 ripe banana, mashed
- 1/4 cup honey or maple syrup
- 1/2 teaspoon vanilla extract
- 1/4 cup chia seeds

- 1/4 cup mini chocolate chips (optional)
- Shredded coconut for rolling (optional)

Instructions:

1. Combine rolled oats, almond butter, mashed banana, honey or maple syrup, vanilla extract, chia seeds, and chocolate chips in a mixing dish.
2. Combine the ingredients well.
3. To make it simpler to handle, chill the mixture for at least 30 minutes.
4. Roll the cooled mixture into bite-sized balls.
5. Roll the energy bites in shredded coconut if preferred for an added layer of flavour.
6. Place in an airtight jar and chill. When you need a fast energy boost, reach for these guilt-free snacks.

Greek Yogurt Parfait with Fresh Berries

Brief Description/Backstory: The Greek Yoghurt Parfait with Fresh Berries is a delicious and healthful snack. This parfait, made with creamy Greek yoghurt, colourful berries, and a touch of honey, will satisfy your sweet need while also supplying antioxidants and probiotics.

Serving Size: 2 parfaits
Prep Time & Cooking Time: 10 minutes

Ingredients:
- 2 cups Greek yogurt
- 1 cup mixed berries (strawberries, blueberries, raspberries)
- 1/4 cup granola
- 2 tablespoons honey
- Fresh mint leaves for garnish

Instructions:
1. Layer Greek yoghurt, mixed berries, and granola in two glasses or bowls.
2. Pour honey over each parfait for extra sweetness.
3. Garnish with fresh mint leaves if desired.
4. Grab a spoon and get into this delectable and nutritious Greek Yoghurt Parfait.

Roasted Chickpeas Three Ways

Brief Description/Backstory:
Roasted Chickpeas Three Ways, a unique spin on a popular food, will revolutionise your snacking habit. Whether you want something savoury, sweet, or spicy, these roasted chickpeas are a crispy and protein-packed snack.

Serving Size: 4
Prep Time & Cooking Time: 40 minutes

Ingredients:
For Savory Chickpeas:
- 2 cans (15 oz each) chickpeas, drained and rinsed
- 2 tablespoons olive oil
- 1 teaspoon garlic powder
- 1 teaspoon smoked paprika
- Salt and pepper to taste
- For Sweet Cinnamon Chickpeas:
- 2 cans (15 oz each) chickpeas, drained and rinsed
- 2 tablespoons coconut oil, melted
- 2 tablespoons maple syrup
- 1 teaspoon ground cinnamon

- 1/4 teaspoon nutmeg
- Pinch of salt
- For Spicy Sriracha Chickpeas:
- 2 cans (15 oz each) chickpeas, drained and rinsed
- 2 tablespoons olive oil
- 2 tablespoons Sriracha sauce
- 1 teaspoon smoked paprika
- Salt to taste

Instructions:
1. Preheat the oven to 400 degrees Fahrenheit (200 degrees Celsius) and line a baking sheet with parchment paper.
2. With a paper towel, carefully dry the chickpeas.
3. Divide the chickpeas into three dishes, one for each flavour.
4. To make savoury chickpeas, combine olive oil, garlic powder, smoked paprika, salt, and pepper in a mixing bowl.
5. Spread out on a baking sheet.
6. To make sweet cinnamon chickpeas, combine melted coconut oil, maple syrup, ground cinnamon, nutmeg, and a touch of salt in a mixing bowl.

7. Spread out on a baking sheet.

8. To make spicy Sriracha chickpeas, combine olive oil, Sriracha sauce, smoked paprika, and salt in a mixing bowl.

9. Spread out on a baking sheet.

10. Roast chickpeas for 30-35 minutes, tossing every 15 minutes to ensure even crisping.

11. Allow to cool before serving these three delectable roasted chickpea varieties.

Avocado and Tomato Salsa with Whole-Grain Chips

Brief Description/Backstory: Enjoy a refreshing bowl of Avocado and Tomato Salsa with whole-grain chips. This snacking pleasure blends creamy avocado, juicy tomatoes, and zesty lime juice, providing a delightful and healthy solution for those looking for a flavour burst without sacrificing health.

Serving Size: 4
Prep Time & Cooking Time: 15 minutes

Ingredients:

- 2 avocados, diced
- 1 cup cherry tomatoes, diced
- 1/4 cup red onion, finely chopped
- 1/4 cup fresh cilantro, chopped
- 1 jalapeño, seeded and minced (optional for heat)
- Juice of 2 limes
- Salt and pepper to taste
- Whole-grain tortilla chips for serving

Instructions:

1. Combine diced avocados, cherry tomatoes, red onion, chopped cilantro, and minced jalapeo in a mixing bowl.
2. Squeeze fresh lime juice over the salad and gently toss to coat.
3. Season to taste with salt and pepper.
4. For a tasty appetiser, serve the Avocado and Tomato Salsa with whole-grain tortilla chips.

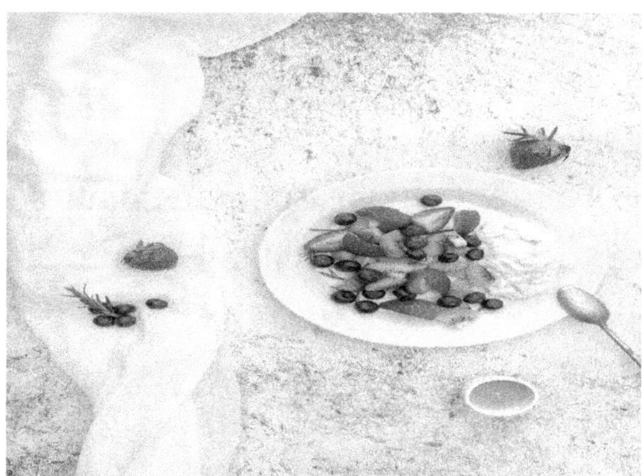

Baked Sweet Potato Fries with Greek Yogurt Dip

Brief Description/Backstory: Baked Sweet Potato Fries with a luscious Greek Yoghurt Dip will elevate your munching experience. These crispy, seasoned fries are not only a guilt-free alternative to typical fries, but they also provide a healthful dose of vitamins and fibre, supplemented with a protein-packed yoghurt dip.

Serving Size: 4
Prep Time & Cooking Time: 30 minutes

Ingredients:
For Sweet Potato Fries:
- 4 medium sweet potatoes, cut into fries
- 2 tablespoons olive oil
- 1 teaspoon paprika
- 1/2 teaspoon garlic powder
- 1/2 teaspoon cumin
- Salt and pepper to taste

For Greek Yogurt Dip:
- 1 cup Greek yogurt
- 1 tablespoon fresh lemon juice

- 1 tablespoon chopped fresh dill
- Salt and pepper to taste

Instructions:

1. Preheat the oven to 425 degrees Fahrenheit (220 degrees Celsius) and line a baking sheet with parchment paper.
2. Toss sweet potato fries with olive oil, paprika, garlic powder, cumin, salt, and pepper in a mixing bowl until equally covered.
3. Arrange the fries on the baking pan in a single layer.
4. Bake the fries for 20-25 minutes, rotating halfway through, until golden and crispy.
5. While the fries are baking, make the dip by combining Greek yoghurt, fresh lemon juice, chopped dill, salt, and pepper.
6. Serve the Baked Sweet Potato Fries alongside the cool Greek Yoghurt Dip.

Quinoa and Black Bean Stuffed Mini Peppers

Brief Description/Backstory: Quinoa and Black Bean Stuffed Mini Peppers are a delicious snack that blends protein-packed quinoa, fiber-rich black beans, and a mix of spices. These bite-sized stuffed peppers are not only tasty but also nutritious, keeping you energised.

Serving Size: 6
Prep Time & Cooking Time: 25 minutes

Ingredients:
1. 12 mini bell peppers, halved and seeds removed
2. 1 cup cooked quinoa
3. 1/2 cup black beans, drained and rinsed
4. 1/2 cup corn kernels (fresh or frozen)
5. 1/4 cup red onion, finely chopped
6. 1 teaspoon ground cumin
7. 1 teaspoon chili powder
8. Salt and pepper to taste
9. Fresh cilantro for garnish

Instructions:

1. Preheat the oven to 375 degrees Fahrenheit (190 degrees Celsius).
2. Combine cooked quinoa, black beans, corn, red onion, ground cumin, chilli powder, salt and pepper in a mixing bowl.
3. Fill each half of a tiny bell pepper with the quinoa and black bean mixture.
4. Bake the stuffed tiny peppers for 15-18 minutes, or until the peppers are soft.
5. Garnish with fresh cilantro and serve these Quinoa and Black Bean Stuffed Mini Peppers as a filling and healthful snack.

Hummus and Veggie Snack Board

Brief Description/Backstory: Create a visually appealing and nutritious snack with a Hummus and Veggie Snack Board. This customizable board features a variety of colorful vegetables, paired with creamy hummus for dipping. Enjoy a satisfying and balanced snacking experience that is rich in vitamins, minerals, and fiber.

Serving Size: 4

Prep Time: 15 minutes

Ingredients:
- 1 cup hummus (store-bought or homemade)
- Baby carrots
- Cherry tomatoes
- Cucumber slices
- Bell pepper strips (assorted colors)
- Sugar snap peas
- Radishes, sliced
- Broccoli florets
- Whole-grain pita bread, cut into triangles

Instructions:
1. On a big serving board or tray, arrange a variety of veggies and pita bread.
2. In the centre of the board, place a bowl of hummus.
3. Arrange the veggies in a pleasing pattern around the hummus bowl.
4. Dip the veggies and pita bread into the creamy hummus to encourage munching.

Apple and Almond Butter Sandwiches

Brief Description/Backstory: Apple and Almond Butter Sandwiches are a healthy and tasty alternative to usual snacking. Crisp apple slices sandwiched between creamy almond butter make for a delectable mix of flavours and textures, making this snack both enjoyable and healthful.

Serving Size: 2
Prep Time: 10 minutes

Ingredients:
- 1 large apple, cored and sliced into rounds
- Almond butter
- Granola (optional)
- Cinnamon (optional)

Instructions:
1. Remove the core from the apple and slice it into rounds.
2. On half of the apple slices, spread a thick amount of almond butter.
3. Sprinkle granola and cinnamon over the almond butter if preferred.

4. To make "sandwiches," top each almond butter-covered apple slice with another apple slice.
5. For a naturally sweet and fulfilling snack, try these Apple and Almond Butter Sandwiches.

Green Smoothie Bowl

Brief Description/Backstory: A Green Smoothie Bowl is a bright and nutrient-dense snack that blends the benefits of leafy greens, fruits, and superfoods. This delicious dish not only fulfils your snack desires but also gives an antioxidant and vitamin boost.

Serving Size: 1
Prep Time: 10 minutes

Ingredients:
- 1 cup spinach or kale, fresh or frozen
- 1/2 frozen banana
- 1/2 cup frozen mango chunks
- 1/2 avocado
- 1/2 cup almond milk

Toppings:

- sliced kiwi,
- chia seeds,
- granola, and coconut flakes

Instructions:
1. Blend spinach or kale, frozen banana, frozen mango pieces, avocado, and almond milk in a blender.
2. Blend until smooth and creamy, adding additional almond milk as required to get the desired consistency.
3. Fill a bowl halfway with the green smoothie.
4. To add texture and flavour, top with sliced kiwi, chia seeds, granola, and coconut flakes.
5. This Green Smoothie Bowl is a nutritious and vivid snack.

Trail Mix with a Twist

Brief Description/Backstory: Add a twist to the typical trail mix by mixing nuts, seeds, dried fruits, and a hint of dark chocolate for a snack that satisfies both sweet and savoury desires. This Trail Mix with a Twist is ideal for on-the-go snacking since it has a good combination of nutrition and energy.

Serving Size: 4
Prep Time: 5 minutes

Ingredients:
- 1 cup mixed nuts (almonds, cashews, walnuts)
- 1/2 cup pumpkin seeds
- 1/2 cup dried cranberries
- 1/4 cup dark chocolate chips or chunks
- 1/4 cup coconut flakes

Instructions:
1. Combine mixed nuts, pumpkin seeds, dried cranberries, dark chocolate chips, and coconut flakes in a mixing dish.
2. Toss the ingredients together until evenly distributed.
3. Divide the trail mix into tiny snack-size bags for easy, portion-controlled munching.
4. Keep our Trail Mix with a Twist on hand for a fast and enjoyable snack whenever and wherever you need it.

CHAPTER 7: INDULGING IN DESSERTS WITHOUT AGING

Dark Chocolate Avocado Mousse

Brief Description/Backstory: Savour the rich and velvety taste of Dark Chocolate Avocado Mousse, a decadent dessert that also happens to be nutritious. The creamy smoothness comes from ripe avocados, providing a delightful pleasure without sacrificing health.

Serving Size: 4
Prep Time & Cooking Time: 15 minutes (plus chilling time)

Ingredients:
- 2 ripe avocados, peeled and pitted
- 1/2 cup dark cocoa powder
- 1/2 cup maple syrup or honey
- 1/4 cup almond milk
- 1 teaspoon vanilla extract

- A pinch of sea salt

Instructions:
1. Combine avocados, dark chocolate powder, maple syrup or honey, almond milk, vanilla extract, and a sprinkling of sea salt in a blender or food processor.
2. Blend the contents until it is smooth and creamy.
3. Pour the mousse into individual serving glasses or bowls.
4. Refrigerate the mousse for at least 2 hours to allow it to firm.
5. Before serving, garnish with shaved dark chocolate or fresh berries.
6. Dark Chocolate Avocado Mousse is a guilt-free indulgence.

Berry Chia Seed Pudding Parfait

Backstory/Brief Description: Enjoy the lightness of a Berry Chia Seed Pudding Parfait, a dessert that combines nutrient-rich chia seed pudding with vivid berries. This parfait not only satisfies your sweet craving but also contains antioxidants and omega-3 fatty acids for an anti-aging treat.

Serving Size: 2
Prep Time & Cooking Time: 10 minutes (plus chilling time)

Ingredients:
For Chia Seed Pudding:
- 1/4 cup chia seeds
- 1 cup almond milk
- 1 tablespoon maple syrup or honey
- 1/2 teaspoon vanilla extract

For Parfait:
- 1 cup mixed berries (strawberries, blueberries, raspberries)
- Granola for layering

Instructions:
1. Whisk together chia seeds, almond milk, maple syrup or honey, and vanilla essence in a container.
2. Allow the chia seed pudding to thicken in the refrigerator for at least 4 hours or overnight.

3. Layer the pudding in serving glasses or bowls with mixed berries and granola after it has set.
4. Repeat the layering until the glasses are completely full.
5. Top with more berries and granola.
6. Serve this Berry Chia Seed Pudding Parfait as a light and healthy dessert.

Banana and Walnut Baked Oatmeal Cups

Brief Description/Backstory: Banana and Walnut Baked Oatmeal Cups are a warm and cosy dish. Individually portioned sweets sweetened with ripe bananas and studded with heart-healthy walnuts for a balanced and delightful dessert experience.

Serving Size: 6 cups
Prep Time & Cooking Time: 30 minutes

Ingredients:
- 2 ripe bananas, mashed
- 2 cups rolled oats

- 1/2 cup chopped walnuts
- 1 teaspoon baking powder
- 1/2 teaspoon cinnamon
- 1/4 teaspoon salt
- 1 cup almond milk
- 1/4 cup maple syrup
- 1 egg
- 1 teaspoon vanilla extract

Instructions:

1. Preheat the oven to 350°F (180°C) and coat a muffin pan with cooking spray.
2. Combine mashed bananas, rolled oats, chopped walnuts, baking powder, cinnamon, and salt in a mixing dish.
3. Whisk together almond milk, maple syrup, egg, and vanilla extract in a separate dish.
4. Pour the wet components into the dry ingredients and incorporate thoroughly.
5. Divide the mixture evenly between the muffin cups.
6. Bake for 20-25 minutes, or until the tops are golden brown and a toothpick inserted comes out clean.
7. Before serving, let the Banana and Walnut Baked Oatmeal Cups to cool slightly.

8. Enjoy these delicious and nutritious muesli cups as a guilt-free dessert.

Coconut and Mango Chia Seed Popsicles

Brief Description/Backstory: Coconut and Mango Chia Seed Popsicles are a tropical treat that blends creamy coconut milk, juicy mango chunks, and the texture of chia seeds. These popsicles are a pleasant treat that is ideal for hot days.

Serving Size: 6 popsicles
Prep Time & Freezing Time: 10 minutes (plus freezing time)

Ingredients:
- 1 cup coconut milk
- 1 cup mango chunks (fresh or frozen)
- 2 tablespoons chia seeds
- 2 tablespoons maple syrup or honey
- 1/2 teaspoon vanilla extract

Instructions:

1. Blend together coconut milk, mango chunks, chia seeds, maple syrup or honey, and vanilla essence in a blender.
2. Blend until completely smooth.
3. Fill popsicle moulds halfway with the mixture.
4. Freeze for at least 4 hours, or until completely frozen.
5. To release the popsicles, run the moulds under warm water.
6. For a guilt-free treat, indulge in the exotic flavours of Coconut and Mango Chia Seed Popsicles.

Almond Flour Blueberry Muffins

Brief Description/Backstory: Almond Flour Blueberry Muffins, a gluten-free and nutrient-rich dessert choice, will satisfy your sweet need. These muffins are baked with almond flour for a soft and supple texture, and they're packed with luscious blueberries for an antioxidant boost.

Serving Size: 12 muffins

Prep Time & Cooking Time: 25 minutes

Ingredients:
- 2 cups almond flour
- 1/2 cup coconut flour
- 1 teaspoon baking powder
- 1/2 teaspoon baking soda
- 1/4 teaspoon salt
- 3 large eggs
- 1/2 cup almond milk
- 1/4 cup melted coconut oil
- 1/4 cup maple syrup or honey
- 1 teaspoon vanilla extract
- 1 cup fresh or frozen blueberries

Instructions:
1. Preheat the oven to 350 degrees Fahrenheit (180 degrees Celsius) and line a muffin pan with paper liners.
2. Whisk together almond flour, coconut flour, baking powder, baking soda, and salt in a large mixing basin.
3. Whisk together the eggs, almond milk, melted coconut oil, maple syrup or honey, and vanilla extract in a separate dish.

4. Pour the wet ingredients into the dry ingredients and stir until just mixed.
5. Fold in the blueberries gently.
6. Divide the batter among the muffin cups in an equal layer.
7. Bake for 18-22 minutes, or until a toothpick inserted comes out clean.
8. Allow the Almond Flour Blueberry Muffins to cool completely before serving this delicious gluten-free dessert.

Greek Yogurt and Honey Parfait with Pistachios

Brief Description/Backstory: Indulge in a dessert that mixes the richness of Greek yoghurt with the sweetness of honey and the crunch of pistachios. This Greek Yoghurt and Honey Parfait with Pistachios is not only tasty, but it's also high in protein and healthy fats, making it a guilt-free dessert.

Serving Size: 2
Prep Time: 10 minutes

Ingredients:

- 2 cups Greek yogurt
- 4 tablespoons honey
- 1/2 cup pistachios, chopped
- Fresh mint leaves for garnish

Instructions:

1. Layer Greek yoghurt in two glasses or bowls and sprinkle honey over each layer.
2. Continue to layer until the glasses are nearly filled.
3. Garnish with chopped pistachios and fresh mint leaves.
4. For a simple yet delectable dessert, serve the Greek Yoghurt and Honey Parfait with Pistachios.

Pumpkin Spice Baked Apples

Brief Description/Backstory: Pumpkin Spice Baked Apples are a delicious way to enjoy the warm and comforting flavours of fall. This dish mixes crisp apples with pumpkin, spices, and a hint of sweetness, resulting in a wonderful treat that captures the essence of the season.

Serving Size: 4
Prep Time & Cooking Time: 30 minutes

Ingredients:
- 4 large apples, cored
- 1/2 cup pumpkin puree
- 2 tablespoons maple syrup
- 1 teaspoon pumpkin spice
- 1/4 cup chopped pecans
- 1/4 cup raisins

Instructions:
1. Preheat the oven to 375°F (190°C) and coat a baking dish with cooking spray.
2. Combine pumpkin puree, maple syrup, pumpkin spice, chopped pecans, and raisins in a mixing bowl.
3. Leave the bottoms of the apples intact to make a well.
4. Fill the pumpkin mixture inside each apple.
5. Cover the baking dish with foil once the apples have been loaded.

6. Bake for 20 minutes, then uncover and continue baking for another 10 minutes, or until the apples are soft.
7. Serve these Pumpkin Spice Baked Apples warm, topped with a dollop of Greek yoghurt or a sprinkling of cinnamon if desired.

Chocolate-Dipped Strawberries with Almonds

Brief Description/Backstory: Add a healthy twist to the classic pairing of chocolate and strawberries. The antioxidant-rich dark chocolate and crunchy almonds in these Chocolate-Dipped Strawberries with Almonds provide a guilt-free pleasure that fulfils your sweet desires.

Serving Size: 12 strawberries
Prep Time & Cooking Time: 20 minutes (plus chilling time)

Ingredients:
- 12 fresh strawberries, washed and dried

- 1/2 cup dark chocolate, melted
- 1/4 cup sliced almonds, toasted

Instructions:
1. Line a baking sheet with parchment paper.
2. Melt dark chocolate in a heatproof dish over a double boiler or in 20-second increments in the microwave.
3. Dip each strawberry into the melted chocolate, coating it well.
4. Place the dipped strawberries on the prepared tray.
5. Over the chocolate-covered strawberries, scatter toasted sliced almonds.
6. Refrigerate for at least 30 minutes, or until the chocolate has set.
7. Chocolate-Dipped Strawberries with Almonds make a delicious and healthful dessert.

Lemon Blueberry Chia Seed Pudding

Brief Description/Backstory: Lemon Blueberry Chia Seed Pudding—a zesty and refreshing alternative that mixes the tanginess of lemon with the sweetness of blueberries—will brighten your dessert experience. This dish will not only satisfy your sweet craving but will also provide you with fibre and omega-3 fatty acids.

Serving Size: 4
Prep Time & Setting Time: 10 minutes (plus chilling time)

Ingredients:
For Chia Seed Pudding:
- 1/4 cup chia seeds
- 1 cup almond milk
- 2 tablespoons maple syrup
- Zest of 1 lemon
- 1/2 teaspoon vanilla extract

For Topping:
- 1 cup fresh blueberries
- Lemon slices for garnish

Instructions:
1. Whisk together the chia seeds, almond milk, maple syrup, lemon zest, and vanilla extract in a mixing dish.

2. Refrigerate the chia seed pudding for at least 4 hours or overnight, or until it achieves a pudding-like consistency.
3. When the chia seed pudding has set, pour it into serving glasses or bowls.
4. Garnish with fresh blueberries and lemon wedges.
5. As a light and tasty dessert, serve this Lemon Blueberry Chia Seed Pudding.

Mango Coconut Rice Pudding

Brief Description/Backstory:
Mango Coconut Rice Pudding will transport your taste senses to the tropics, combining the richness of ripe mango with the smoothness of coconut-infused rice pudding. Enjoy this tropical pleasure without fear of jeopardising your health.

Serving Size: 6
Prep Time & Cooking Time: 40 minutes

Ingredients:
- 1 cup Arborio rice

- 1 can (14 oz) coconut milk
- 2 cups almond milk
- 1/2 cup maple syrup
- 1 teaspoon vanilla extract
- Pinch of salt
- 2 ripe mangoes, peeled and diced
- Toasted coconut flakes for garnish

Instructions:
1. Combine Arborio rice, coconut milk, almond milk, maple syrup, vanilla essence, and a touch of salt in a saucepan.
2. Over medium heat, bring the mixture to a simmer, stirring regularly.
3. Reduce the heat to low and continue to cook for 30-35 minutes, or until the rice is tender and the custard is creamy.
4. Remove from the heat and set aside to cool somewhat.
5. Fold in the sliced mangoes gently.
6. Serve the Mango Coconut Rice Pudding in bowls.
7. To enhance texture and flavour, garnish with toasted coconut flakes.
8. Without ageing, enjoy the tropical deliciousness of this delicacy.

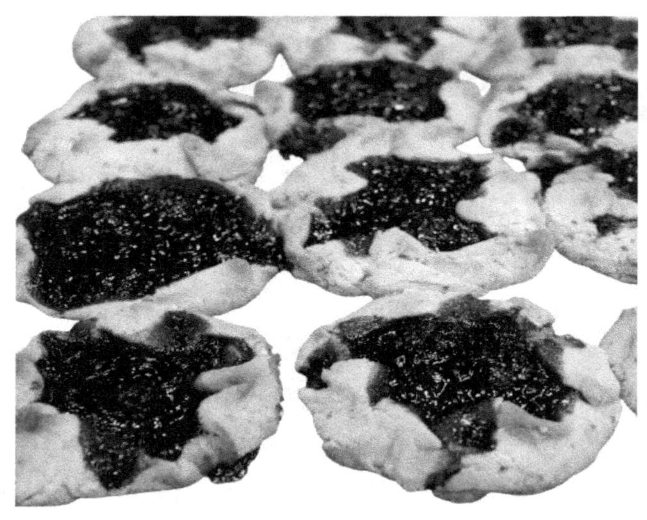

CHAPTER 8:

Welcome to Forever Young Entertaining, a place where the art of feeding your guests delectable, health-conscious dishes meets the joy of hosting. In this section, we dive into the domain of facilitating Sound Supper Gatherings, furnishing you with master ways to find some kind of harmony among extravagance and supplement thickness. Moreover, we'll uncover the insider facts behind making Mark Mixed drinks that entice the taste buds as well as proposition a healthful lift, guaranteeing that your social occasions are significant, energetic, and age-resisting.

Area 1: Facilitating Solid Supper Gatherings

Eating with a Reason

Leave on a culinary excursion that celebrates both flavor and prosperity. Facilitating a Solid Supper Gathering is a fine art, and inside these pages, you'll find tips and deceives to organize a menu that charms the sense of taste while supporting wellbeing. From tidbits to treats, figure out how to mix supplement rich fixings into each dish without settling on taste. Make your dinner parties an experience that engages the senses and supports a Forever Young lifestyle by exploring inventive plate and presentation methods.

Area 2: Discover the art of balance with our expert advice

for balancing indulgences and nutrient density Mastering the Art of Moderation Indulgence and nutrient density do not have to be at odds. We dig into the study of part control, offering experiences on making a menu that permits visitors to enjoy each chomp without the substantialness of overabundance. From picking the right cooking techniques to integrating a rainbow of leafy foods, these tips guarantee that your evening gatherings are both luxurious and wellbeing cognizant. Raise your facilitating game as you strike the ideal balance among wantonness and sustenance.

Area 3: Signature Mixed drinks with a Wholesome Lift

Making Elixirs of Essentialness

Raise your glass to Mark Mixed drinks that go past simple drinks — they become elixirs of imperativeness. In this segment, we reveal recipes for mixed drinks that entice the taste buds as well as proposition a dietary punch. These cocktails, which are intended to complement your Forever Young lifestyle, include fruit infusions that are high in antioxidants and herbal infusions. Learn how to transform the bar into a wellness haven where each drink contributes to a healthier lifestyle.

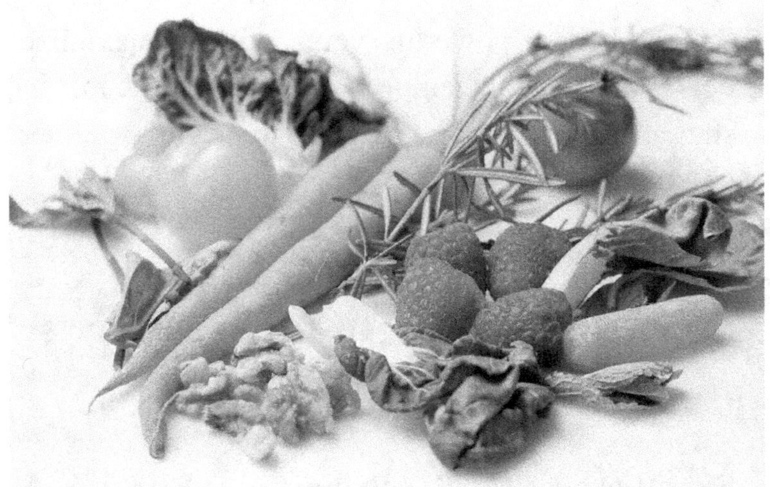

CHAPTER 9: FITNESS FUEL: PRE AND POST-WORKOUT NUTRITION

Leave on an excursion of ideal wellness with Chapter 9, where we investigate the vital job of nourishment in your pre and post-gym routine schedules. Release the capability of your exercises with power-stuffed pre-exercise feasts, find recuperation tidbits that upgrade your outcomes, and dive into hydration hacks intended for dynamic ways of life. In this section, we disentangle the science behind powering your body for maximized operation, guaranteeing that each rep, step, and stretch carries you nearer to your wellness objectives.

Segment 1: Power-Stuffed Pre-Exercise Dinners

Empowering Your Excursion

Get ready to overcome your wellness routine with a complete manual for Power-Stuffed Pre-Exercise Dinners. In this part, we reveal an assortment of healthfully thick recipes that fuel your body with the energy it needs for ideal execution. From protein-rich morning meals to sugar stacked snacks, get familiar with the specialty of timing and arrangement to expand your exercise potential. Express farewell to weakness and hi to supported energy as you find the ideal equilibrium of supplements to launch your wellness process.

Segment 2: Recuperation Snacks for Ideal Outcomes

Rejuvenate and Recharge

Open the privileged insights of compelling recuperation with our manual for post-exercise sustenance. Whether you're taking part in strength preparing, cardio, or a mix of both, legitimate recuperation is vital to accomplishing ideal outcomes. Plunge into a determination of Recuperation Bites intended to renew glycogen stores, fix muscle tissues, and lessen post-practice irritation. Find the ideal proportion of protein, carbs, and fundamental supplements to help your body's recuperation cycle, guaranteeing you return quickly more grounded after each exercise.

Segment 3: Hydration Hacks for Dynamic Ways of life

Extinguishing Your Hunger for Progress

Hydration is the uncelebrated yet truly great individual of any wellness venture, and in this part, we uncover Hydration Hacks custom fitted for dynamic ways of life. Get familiar with the significance of remaining sufficiently hydrated previously, during, and after your exercises. From injected water recipes to electrolyte-rich refreshments, find how appropriate hydration can upgrade your perseverance, further develop recuperation, and add to generally prosperity. Release the force of hydration and lift your wellness game with these reviving and intentional drink decisions.

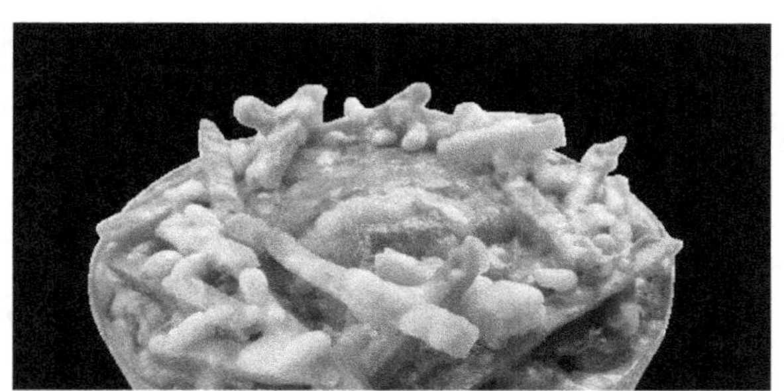

CHAPTER 10: STAYING FOREVER YOUNG ON THE GO

In the speedy cadence of life, keeping an Eternity Youthful way of life isn't just reachable yet can likewise be unimaginably fulfilling. Chapter 10 is your manual for "Remaining Perpetually Youthful in a hurry," offering bits of knowledge into good dieting while at the same time voyaging, pursuing shrewd decisions at eateries and cheap food outlets, and guaranteeing you have the ideal convenient snacks for any experience. Plunge into this section to find the specialty of supporting your body, in any event, when you're continually progressing.

Segment 1: Smart dieting While at the same time Voyaging

Health Past Boundaries

Leave on an excursion that rises above topographical limits while focusing on your prosperity. " Good dieting While at the same time Voyaging" unwinds the key to keeping up with your Eternity Youthful way of life, no matter what your area. From useful ways to pack nutritious snacks to unraveling café menus, figure out how to settle on careful food decisions that line up with your wellbeing objectives. Whether you're on an excursion, traveling to another objective, or investigating unknown regions, this segment guarantees that your culinary experiences supplement your obligation to remaining Perpetually Youthful.

Area 2: Shrewd Decisions at Cafés and Cheap Food Outlets

Translating the Menu Labyrinth

Eating out doesn't need to wreck your Eternity Youthful excursion. " The book "Smart Choices at Restaurants and Fast Food Outlets" gives you the knowledge you need to confidently navigate menus. Learn how to decipher portion sizes, identify nutrient-dense options, and make well-informed choices that are in line with your health-conscious lifestyle. This section gives you the ability to dine out without compromising your commitment to staying Forever Young at any establishment, from fine dining establishments to quick-service restaurants.

Area 3: Fueling Your Active Lifestyle with "Portable Snacks for Any Adventure"

"Portable Snacks for Any Adventure" makes sure you have the right food to keep you going whether you're on the go, hiking, or just commuting. Take a look at a carefully selected selection of healthy snacks that are also easy to carry. From custom made energy bars to trail blend varieties, figure out how to make a versatile storage space that upholds your Eternity Youthful objectives, making each experience a very much energized and fulfilling experience.

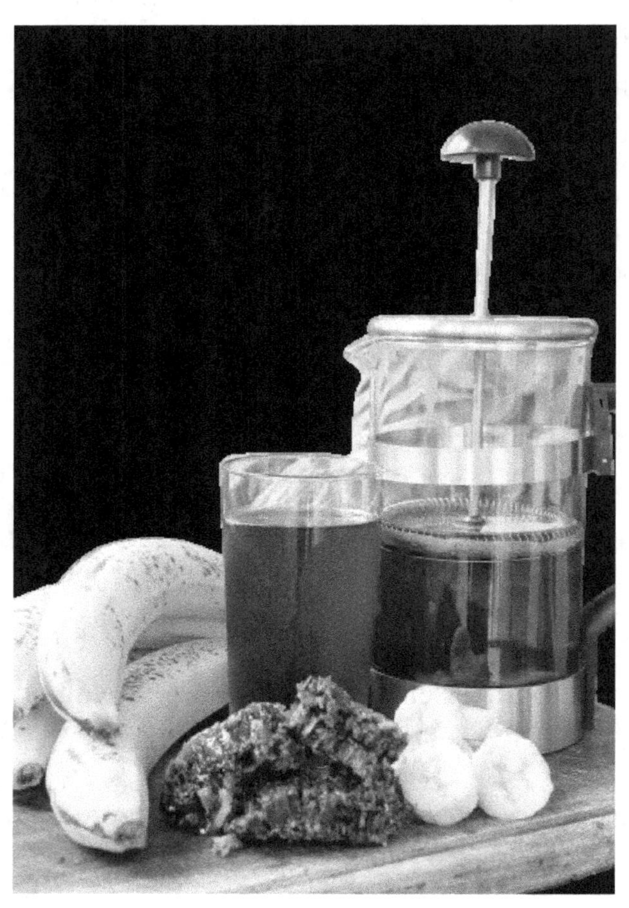

CONCLUSIONS

Additional Resources for the Forever Young Diet

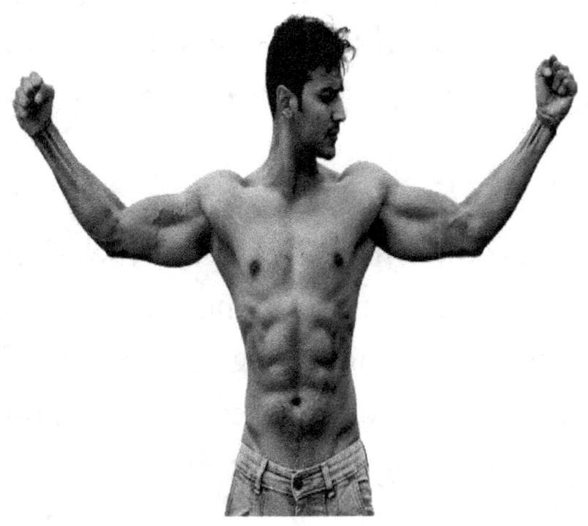

Setting out on the Eternity Youthful Eating routine isn't simply a culinary experience; it's a comprehensive way of life change pointed toward challenging age and encouraging ideal prosperity. To supplement the insight found in the Eternity Youthful Eating regimen Cookbook, a variety of extra assets anticipates, offering support, local area commitment, and continuous training for those focused on the quest for never-ending imperativeness.

Online Community Forum: Associate with close allies on the committed Everlastingly Youthful Living Web-based Local area Gathering. This computerized space fills in as a center point for people sharing their encounters, wins, and difficulties on the Eternity Youthful excursion. Participate in conversations, look for counsel, and fashion associations with similar fans who figure out the subtleties of embracing a young driven way of life.

Forever Young Living Blog: Dig into the rich woven artwork of content on the authority Always Youthful Living Site. The blog is a great source of information and inspiration, with in-depth articles on the science behind anti-aging nutrition and inspiring success stories from people whose lives have changed. Keep up to date with the most recent examination, patterns, and master bits of knowledge to intensify how you might interpret the Eternity Youthful standards.

Interactive Meal Planner:
Tailor your Eternity Youthful involvement in the assistance of an Intelligent Feast Organizer. In addition to the Forever Young Diet Cookbook, this

dynamic tool helps you create individualized meal plans that are in line with your dietary preferences and health objectives. Easily integrate the cookbook's standards into your day to day daily practice with this easy to understand organizer.

Exclusive Webinars and Workshops:
Extend your insight through selective online classes and studios facilitated by specialists in sustenance, wellness, and comprehensive prosperity. These live occasions give an intuitive stage to acquiring further bits of knowledge into the Eternity Youthful way of thinking. Engage with professionals, take part in Q&A sessions, and learn useful health-enhancing advice.

Podcast Series – Forever Young Insights:
Submerge yourself in the Eternity Youthful Bits of knowledge webcast series, where charming conversations unfurl around different parts of a young driven way of life. Check out interviews with wellbeing specialists, accounts of individual changes, and investigations of the comprehensive methodology supported by the Eternity Youthful Eating regimen. Allow this to digital broadcast be

your hear-able aide on your excursion to imperishable living.

Recipe App: The Forever Young Recipe App can take your culinary experience to the next level. This helpful application gives fast and advantageous admittance to a broad assortment of restoring recipes. Peruse classes, save your #1 dishes, and easily make shopping records to smooth out your dinner planning. The application is a down to earth ally for incorporating the cookbook's standards into your day to day existence.

Monthly Challenges: Infuse a component of tomfoolery and inspiration into your Eternity Youthful excursion with Month to month Difficulties. These difficulties, spreading over nourishment, wellness, and care, are intended to unite the local area in shared objectives. Keep tabs on your development, praise accomplishments, and cultivate a feeling of kinship w